Peeling Back the Onion on Prostate Cancer

Peeling Back the Onion on Prostate Cancer

Darnell Shaw

This book is not intended as a substitute for the medical advice of physicians. The reader should consult a physician regularly in any matters relating to his/her health, particularly with respect to any symptoms or illness that may require diagnosis or medical attention.

Copyright © 2024 by Darnell Shaw

All rights reserved. No part of this book may be reproduced or transmitted in any form or by any means, electronic or mechanical, including photocopying, recording, or any information storage and retrieval system, without permission in writing from the author.

ISBN: 978-1-6653-0917-2 – Paperback
eISBN: 978-1-6653-0918-9 – eBook

These ISBNs are the property of BookLogix for the express purpose of sales and distribution of this title. The content of this book is the property of the copyright holder only. BookLogix does not hold any ownership of the content of this book and is not liable in any way for the materials contained within. The views and opinions expressed in this book are the property of the Author/Copyright holder, and do not necessarily reflect those of BookLogix.

Library of Congress Control Number: 2024924697

☉This paper meets the requirements of ANSI/NISO Z39.48-1992 (Permanence of Paper)

1 1 1 8 2 4

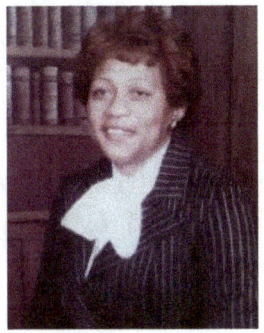 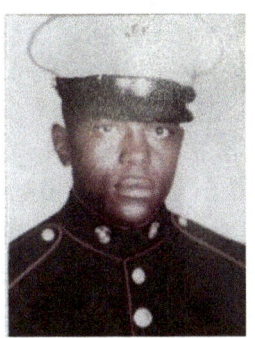

Beulah Shaw   *James Harrell*

This Book is dedicated to my late mother, Mrs. Beulah M. Shaw, and my brother James E. Harrell, a Marine and Army veteran, who fought a good fight of faith. Why? My mother, Mrs. Shaw, is responsible for me being the man I am today through her pouring and teaching me knowledge, understanding, and, most of all, wisdom. She always said, "The best is yet to come." She stressed not to be anybody's fool—a poor fool, young fool, rich fool, church fool, or stupid fool! She said to be a wise fool! "Gain wisdom, son!"

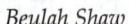

I also include my oldest brother, a great man who served his family and country with honors. He served in the United States Marine Corps at Camp Lejune, North Carolina, and later died at age forty-six from stomach cancer, which metastasized to the prostate. Family, for seven years James was unaware the water he drank and bathed in from 1977 was contaminated with unknown cleaning chemicals.

So, in their memory, I honor and dedicate this book as an instrument to pull humanity back from a dangerous disease, cancer, as it has tried to get the best of humanity for centuries.

Did you know that in 2024, the National Cancer Institute projected that there will be 299,010 new cases of prostate cancer, which equates to 14.9 percent?[1] **Prostate cancer is 14.9 percent of all types of cancer cases.** These statistics are alarming, and our death cases are staggering at 35,250 deaths from prostate cancer, and 5.8 percent for all types of cancer deaths. Our silver lining is we have a 97.5 percent five-year survival rate with early detection, Family.

A Black man is diagnosed every thirteen minutes with prostate cancer, as reported by Zero Prostate Cancer. *Wow!* What an alarming statistic. Let's look at the death rate by race and ethnicity, per one hundred thousand persons. These statistics come from National Cancer Institute's age-adjusted data, 2018–2022. The median age at diagnosis is sixty-seven for all races.

---

[1] The National Cancer Institute, https://www.cancer.gov/prostate

Prostate Death Rate per 100,000 Persons

Death Rate Percentages

All Races	19.0 per
Hispanic	15.4 per
Non-Hispanic American/ Indian/Alaska Native	19.4 per
Asian/Pacific Islander	8.8 per
Black	**37.2 per**
White	18.1 per

Family, let's explore the onion layers for all men and focus on the Black race and see why we are twice as likely to die! Men, are you ready? *"Let's Go!"*

Contents

Foreword
xi
Preface
xiii
Introduction
xvii

Who I Am: The Seed
1

What is a Prostate?
7

Shaw's Victory over Cancer
15

Cancer Diagnosis and Treatment Options
27

Erectile Dysfunction and Mental Struggles
35

Intimacy and Sex
41

Physical Touch Post-Surgery Q&A
45

Acknowledgments
53
Wellness Resources
55

Foreword

I met Darnell in June of 2020, during the height of the COVID-19 pandemic. We met through technology, as is the case for many in this digital age. As we got to know each other, what struck me most about Darnell was his sense of humor and his love of God and people. I eventually realized this was a man I could spend the rest of my life with, and that is what I chose to do. We got married on November 21, 2021.

During our courtship, Darnell shared that he had been diagnosed with prostate cancer years prior to our meeting. He walked me through his cancer journey, from being diagnosed, to treatment, and recovery. Over time, he also revealed the impact that cancer had on other family members as well. I could certainly relate, as I had lost my maternal grandfather and grandmother to different forms of cancer. I could also relate to this as a licensed clinical psychologist who comes alongside clients on their medical journeys.

Although I was not with Darnell during his battle with prostate cancer, I can say that I now get a front-row seat in witnessing the impact of his medical journey. Over the course of our courtship and marriage, I've had the privilege of watching my husband encourage others toward healthy living. His passion is contagious and has personally impacted the way I live my life. I am now a healthier woman because of Darnell's influence. I make healthier lifestyle decisions because of him. It's my expectation that after reading this book, you'll do the same.

Peeling Back the Onion on Prostate Cancer represents the birth of my husband's purpose and passion. It's personal to him. He recognizes the importance of early detection in saving lives and has made it his personal mission to spread the word! As Darnell takes you on this journey, you'll get a bird's eye view of the impact that cancer had on him and his family. You get the opportunity to read a story of triumph over tragedy. And by the time you finish, you'll be educated, equipped, and empowered to live well! Are you ready? Well then, *"Let's go!"*

—Dr. Robin Shaw

Preface

My purpose today, Family, is to share my personal struggles with transparency, putting pride aside. You will experience my pain and victory on my prostate cancer journey. You see, information and knowledge, when used properly, bring wisdom!

This powerful resource was developed using my personal life experiences and talking to several hundred men battling prostate cancer over ten-plus years. The disease is curable. Yes, let me repeat myself: cancer is a big C—*curable* in all men with early detection. [2]Family, did you know 69.4 percent of prostate cancer cases are caught in the first stage?

There are four stages of severity that's used to rate cancer, and the risk goes up the later we start testing our prostate. The good news is, after catching prostate cancer at stage one, it stays localized in the prostate, and the five-year survival rate for prostate cancer goes up to 97.5

---

[2] The National Cancer Institute, https://www.cancer.gov/prostate

percent. Key factors are to get the ball rolling on testing for a starting point. Next is the kind of treatment option you receive, and how each of our unique bodies respond to treatment. Last, Family, is do your own research, and ask for assistance if you suspect you have symptoms with urine flow, pain, or frequent trips to the bathroom at night.

What men must do is know their prostate health status. Prostate cancer is a slow-growing cancer and goes undetected for years without noticeable symptoms. Family, cancer has no respect for the person when it effects a man. It treats all men the same regardless of race or ethnicity.

Later in this book, we will explore "peeling back the onion" on men's prostate health. My use of the onion is metaphoric and symbolic of the circle of life that dates to the Latin meaning "unity or oneness." The onion also connects to prosperity and protection, and in rituals like weddings and funerals, it signifies eternity for its unique layers. It is like the prostate; when you take it apart, two seminal glands, urethra gland passageway, you disrupt the human reproductive system and the life cycle.

We can see only one layer at a time, but underneath—as we get deeper—there are thicker layers on the journey as we get closer to the core of life for the onion and man.

Family, as you walk through this timeline, you will see four brothers who have tackled their cancer diagnosis, and three of the four survived. We have the victory over cancer! All four brothers exercised a strong faith in God as kingdom citizens. We believed and walked by faith knowing the kingdom is now as we saw our healings manifest in pictures or visions by Jesus' example. Living through these monumental life events in the family created a strong passion and desire to work on spreading the good news of the gospel for me. Family, it came with a hefty price, and I felt it deep inside like a sharp stabbing feeling so let me start peeling this onion and share my experiences with you.

I said to myself, "Self, if Jesus got beaten, rocks thrown at him, and was finally crucified on the cross . . ."

"*Yes,*" I replied, "Then he was buried in a borrowed tomb, and on the third day, he got up for me and you. Oh, yes sir! I am special and can do impossible things too."

This is personal, Family, and my mental pain got so bad I started having feelings of doubt and depression and a lot of sleepless nights. This led me to get some mental counseling to address my sleeplessness, as well as medication as needed. I got so angry and pissed off, that I climbed into my cave and shut down from functioning in public. I just felt like withdrawal was the answer to my pain. Not!

Stay with me, Family, as I get deeper into the onion layers and come out of this victoriously. Are you ready? Well, "*Let's Go!*"

Introduction

It is no coincidence that you're about to explore this powerful resource, "a gift" with personal testimonies and self-help aids to assist you, Family, to preserve humanity through the eyes of a Black Kingdom Man of God, Ambassador Darnell Shaw. This journey will carry you through my trials and tribulations, dealing with all aspects of my cancer battle, with transparency. My purpose and critical objective are to educate and encourage all men to get regular prostate health and wellness checks before the recommended age range of forty to fifty. I am suggesting that prostate checks begin at age thirty-five to allow for early detection and corrective measures to save lives. My family health history is an example of how early detection could have saved my big brother's life.

My efforts are to bring a refreshing, magnifying light to an age-old problem through an Ambassador of Christ lens. I believe that together we will manifest tangible actions and change the narrative to increase the lives of all men and especially Black men.

According to the American Cancer Society, one in six African American men will develop prostate cancer, in comparison to one in eight White men. The death rate for Black men with prostate cancer is twice as high compared to White men. We need to focus on identifying causes and implementing steps to close the gap.

My wellness resources, the Prostate Health Card, the Prostate Recorder and Family Medical History Recorder will provide meaningful reminders to get checked early and learn about your health digits and limits sooner. The next goal of this resource is for men to step back from their prideful nature and help each other to *live well, Family.* This approach is best achieved when we stick together and educate one another, even when it's *personal* and *private*. Iron sharpens iron, one man strengthens another man!

Are you ready to walk alongside me and see what the end will be? Ready, set, *"Let's Go!"*

1

Who I Am: The Seed

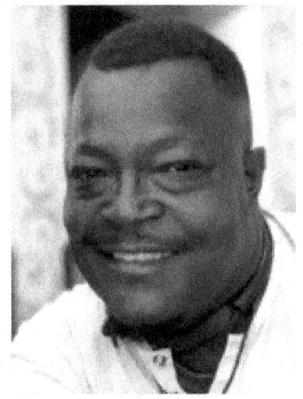

Darnell Shaw

Family, just like an onion seed that enters the ground of the Earth, we are planted in the womb. It's the beginning of life where nurturing occurs, and we receive nutrients for our development.

My story began in Pasquotank County in the township of Elizabeth City, North Carolina, about sixty-five miles east of the Atlantic Ocean. My parents are Mrs. Beulah M. Shaw and Joseph Shaw, Sr. They married and had four strong, healthy, vibrant young boys, active in the community. We were talented boys who got dirty and didn't shy away from anything exciting and daring. Let me paint a picture of how I grew up with my parents by sharing a few personal details to allow you to walk my journey.

My mother was born in Perquimans County, North Carolina, and graduated from P.W. Moore High School. My father was born in Currituck, North Carolina, and graduated from Currituck Union High School.

My Dad and Mom started their new life living in Elizabeth City. The marriage got off to a great start, with one older son James, born in 1953, and three younger boys were born behind each other like a staircase. The next older brother was born in December of 1961, I was born in February of 1963, and my younger brother was born in July of 1964. Looking at the time between ages, my oldest brother and I almost look like we are twins. As we grew up in Elizabeth City, several key things happened that would shape our lives forever and impact who I am today. Several years later, at the beginning of March 1970, we were all shocked by the accidental death of my father, Joseph Shaw Sr. All I could remember was having to face this tragedy at the age of seven as a young boy who highly depended on Dad for his joy, love, and survival. This horrific event changed me for a lifetime.

This layer of the onion is close to my core and the pain penetrated my heart with a scar that required time and years to heal. The next major tragedy was the loss of my mother's mom who raised her after her birth mom passed. Life after that shifted, and we all felt the impact of not having a grandparent at home.

The significance of this is family history for trends. So, an onion layer was lost with the passing of our parents. Back then, family records were mostly known through word of mouth or recorded in the Bible. My father's medical history was gone forever, and we could not reset the clock to know if any major diseases were in his DNA or genes to pass along his health history. My dad worked in all kinds of environments like cleaning jobs, in an automotive repair shop, to assembly lines, at a major automotive factory.

For the next few years, life as we knew it shifted for the entire family, and we tightened up and matured fast, helping where we could and taking care of the household affairs. My life was forever altered as I found myself consumed with an overwhelming sense of sorrow and fury. I navigated through the various stages of grief, each one presenting its unique challenges and obstacles, until I finally arrived at a place of acceptance, which struck me like a sudden brick to the face. *Pow!*

These experiences transformed me in ways I never could have imagined, leaving an indelible mark on my heart and soul. I had to toughen up, bite my tongue, fake smiles, and grit my teeth to cope throughout my childhood and adult life.

Adversity hardened me instead of breaking me to pieces under stress. Having a mother who stood in the gap made all the difference in me continuing to strive as I matured into the person I am today! Soon, I mastered the art of pretending roles in every social setting, and I got through all my classes and significant school events up to graduation from Northern High School in 1981.

. . .

My next move was to get out of town, join the military, get an education, and get into college at Elizabeth City State University (ECSU). My two older brothers set the example for me to try the Army National Guard and possibly Army Reserve Officer Training Camp ROTC. Fast forward with me in time as I share my military experiences after completing Army Basic Training at Fort Benning, Georgia, in 1983. I completed all my required training with honors and came back to my National Guard Unit, the 119th Infantry Unit on fire and highly motivated to lead. As time went on, I tested high on many skills tests and was promoted to an Army Specialist E-4 in my Army National Guard Unit. I had leadership skills, I proved it over time, and was selected to receive a ROTC scholarship at ECSU.

In 1986, I completed Army ROTC as one of the top cadets, was selected as Army 2nd Lieutenant, and was asked to lead the Class of 1986 Military Ceremony for Our Senior Class Graduation. That same year, I was handpicked for hometown recruiting as a Gold Bar College Recruiter for ECSU. As time passed, I took every opportunity seriously and followed the Army's slogan "Be All You Can Be" to my heart by meeting all challenges one hundred percent.

After completing the Infantry Officers Basic Training Camp, I was singled out as an officer to keep an eye on for being focused on getting results with the gift of leadership. I was challenged and selected to attend Airborne School, Ranger School, Pathfinder School and assigned to the 197th Infantry Brigade at Fort Benning, Georgia. At my unit I excelled at all my assignments and was selected to do special missions at the National Training Center in California, and Joint Readiness Training Center in Arkansas. As a Platoon Leader and Company Executive Officer I completed the Expert Infantry Badge training.

The biggest test was to come as America went to war with Iraq in 1990 during Operation Desert Shield. My Brigade and Battalion, the 118th Infantry was tagged to support the 24th Infantry Division with its war mission. My life changed as I experienced lots of traumatic situations while deployed in the Gulf War from 1990 to 1991 Operation Desert Storm. The environment as an Infantry Leader required me to be out front and face many hazards and the enemy face to face. In the desert, I was promoted to Captain and was referred to as "Captain Combat" because of my can-do attitude! On February 24, 1991, the ground campaign started and penetrated deep into Iraq. As soon as it started, American Forces and Allies attacked for the next one hundred hours. Many tragic events happened that made the Gulf War a hell of a pill to swallow as bombs and air attacks went on for seventy-two hours. Our task force had a leading role as the 24th Infantry Division Lead the assault. As days and weeks passed, we collected and captured hundreds of prisoners, equipment, specialized weaponry, and ammunition, deep into Iraq territory.

Before we knew it, our Commander in Chief, and key leaders, sent orders down the chain of command to destroy and burn ammunition and equipment. Burn pits were everywhere and smoke filled the air for miles twenty-four hours a day. Besides the dust blowing deep into our nostrils, we also had hazardous smoke flowing from burning fire all day and throughout the night. Being at war is an onion layer that leaves deep dark emotional scars and marks inside and out pre-combat and post-recover operations. After the smoke and burning stopped, we had to wash-up all our equipment from top to bottom and load things up to redeploy back to the United States.

Upon getting back and looking at our war zone, we were exposed to all kinds of chemicals in the Gulf War that contained cancer-producing agents. Family, another onion mark to scar me for cancer risk we were either oblivious to or didn't know about when we were deployed to Saudia Arabia and Iraq.

Here's the deal I was left with, Family, too many unknowns like undiagnosed illnesses, or abnormal cell formation caused by all kinds of environmental exposures from dirty conditions, grease, grime, and chemical compounds. As time would have it, I came back and received orders to complete the Infantry Officers Advance Course. In 1992, after the Infantry Advance Course, I completed Pathfinder school at Fort Benning, Georgia. I was set up to command an Infantry Company of 130 plus soldiers. After graduation, I was assigned to the 82nd Airborne Division, Fort Bragg, North Carolina. At the 82nd Airborne Division, I was selected to command Alpha Company 3rd Battalion 504th Parachute Infantry Regiment. About two years later, I was selected again to command the Division Headquarters Airborne Leaders Course for specialized training. That's who I am, so, *"Let's Go!"*

2

What is a Prostate?

God created Man in his image to procreate the earth, take dominion of the earth, multiply, and be fruitful. So, I see the prostate as a "seed." The prostate is a mystery to most men, and most don't truly understand its role until something goes wrong in the male reproductive system. What I mean is that men may have problems with the bladder, urine flow, or sexual activity. This translates to sexual performance that prevents or hinders their ability to have an effective sexual life with a woman to have a child.

Let's explore the prostate and peel back a layer of the onion like the skin on this vegetable as we look at the male reproductive organ as a vegetable that has seeds. Just like vegetables have layers, visualize an image of an onion growing in the earth with its roots on the bottom, and green stems extending through the ground. As it grows toward the sunlight, it flowers and produces seeds. The rain and earth nourish and feed the onion until it gets bigger and creates layers or rings of growth over time. As a man ages, we too need the proper nutrients and adequate vitamins to augment the lack nutrients in food processing.

So, Family, in this layer it's mysterious and personal how onions are used in our everyday lives. I will take you through several layers to look at your wellness, and reasons to track your key digits. As a comparison between the two, they both start out as seeds and need ingredients like a healthy environment and adequate attention for growth to full maturity. Man needs, food, water, shelter, sunlight, and sources from this same type of environment along with other plant-like nutrients to mature to adults.

Let's go deeper into the next layer below and explore more details of what happens when the environment negatively impacts layers. We suffer from abnormal attributes that cause problems in the development process for man. Family, just know that any past injuries, internal to your body or external environments, have the potential to create abnormal cell growth for years.

Yes, Family, get all your routine checkups and pay attention to different signs and symptoms your body is showing. Talk to the experts and don't suffer in silence. Family, every two minutes a man is diagnosed with prostate cancer according to Zero Prostate Cancer. Additionally, every seventeen minutes Black men are at risk of dying if not checked by a qualified health care physician. The silent killer that can be prevented. See the image to assist you in knowing more about the prostate location. The key is just go!

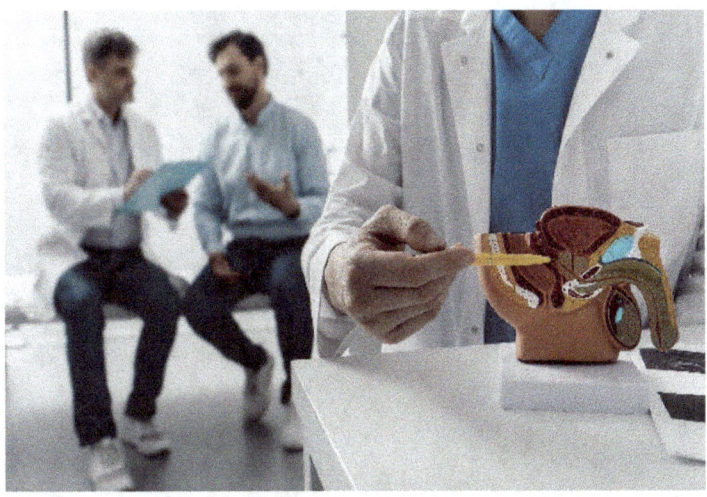

Prostate model and location cross section male anatomy. [3]

The male reproductive system known as the penis, testes, and scrotum has a walnut-sized object called the prostate that I liken to the onion. The prostate surrounds the urethra tube that extends from the exit end of the penis to the bladder, where urine fluid is stored for release. So, you see that it's like an onion with a root on one end and stem.

See the diagram on the next page for the parts of the prostate and bladder and notice that there is the male ejaculatory duct that carries the sperm for reproduction.

---

[3] Image credit: iStock by Getty Images

10 *What is a Prostate?*

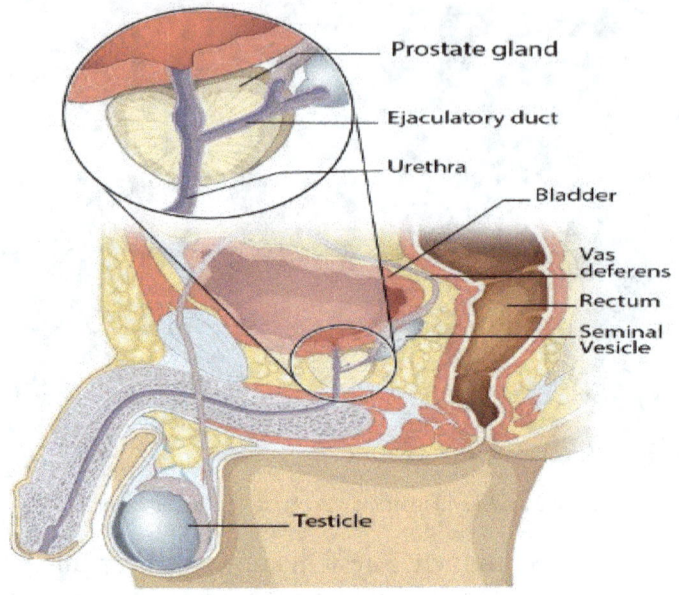

Expanded view of the male prostate gland and duct work.[4]

Another important role of the prostate is to aid the seminal glands in producing sperm and assist the penis with holding an erection.

That all starts from the brain or "control tower." In summary, Family, without getting too deep into the reproductive system, remember that we need the prostate to function and produce sperm to have seeds to start the reproductive process in a woman. The sperm travel from the prostate through the urethra tube into the penis and exit. *No prostate, no sperm, Family. This is a key point you need to know.*

. . .

---

[4] Image credit: Centers for Disease Control and Prevention

Let's explore what makes for a healthy prostate and how to get it checked. I would like to take a wellness approach to educate you on some basic facts about the prostate.

Family, get started with your regular checks at age thirty-five to establish a baseline, but if it runs in your family start earlier. Make sure to also include family history, and problems with cancer diagnosis as key indicators to speed up checks immediately. Please use your medical team, they are experts.

Two methods are used to check the prostate in men once they reach a mature age depending on factors from the urologist community. There are things we can do before we go in for an exam, and the list below will help shed some light on prevention.

- Self-education on prostate role in the body
- Stay active and exercise regularly
- Don't smoke and avoid hazardous environments
- Maintain a healthy weight/diet (consume veggies and fruits)
- Familiarize yourself with how it's checked
- Learn about key diagnosis results or digits
- Read about prevention steps and treatment protocol from a specialized doctor
- Ask other men who you trust

The first is known as a Digital Rectal Exam (DRE) where a qualified medical doctor inserts his lubricated, gloved finger into the anus and manually feels the prostate and examines its size and other characteristics.

See picture below.

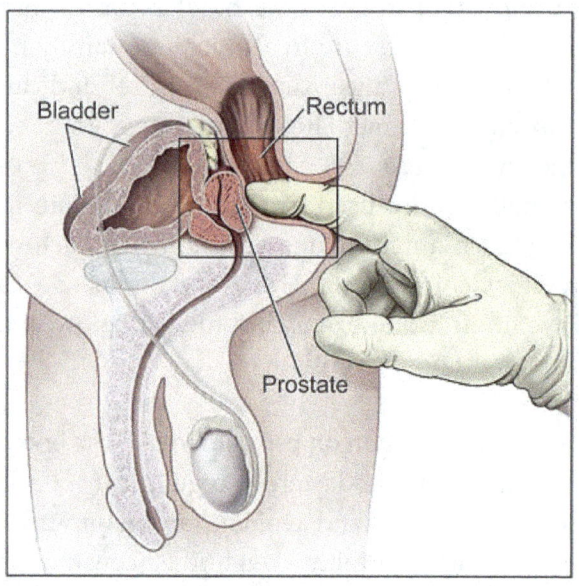

Picture of Digital Rectal Exam (DRE) [5]

An additional approach to screening for prostate cancer is the Prostate-Specific Antigen (PSA) test. A blood sample is drawn from your arm and put into a tube during a standard health check-up. The PSA blood sample is then sent to a medical laboratory for analysis. The resulting numeric value is determined by several factors, such as age, size, symptoms, and risk factors.

---

[5] Image credit: Wikipedia.org, Public Doman.

Family, the key point is to have a health baseline number, the lower the better.

Go get checked! Let "good health be your wealth," as I always say.

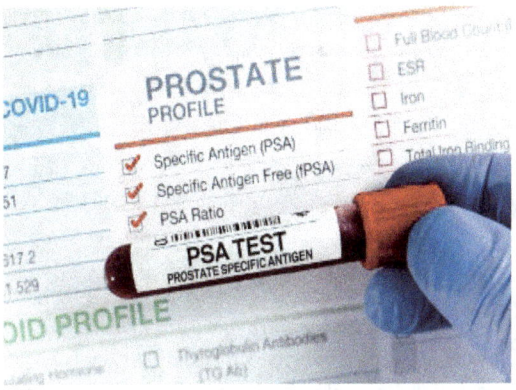

Picture of blood test known as Prostate Specific Antigen (PSA). [6]

Let's talk about prostate symptoms and what you can experience. The picture below shows you some common signs a man can experience in his lifetime. It's very important not to overlook these signs and have your doctor or urologist check you as early as possible.

---

[6] Image credit: PSA Tulsa Procedures™

14 *What is a Prostate?*

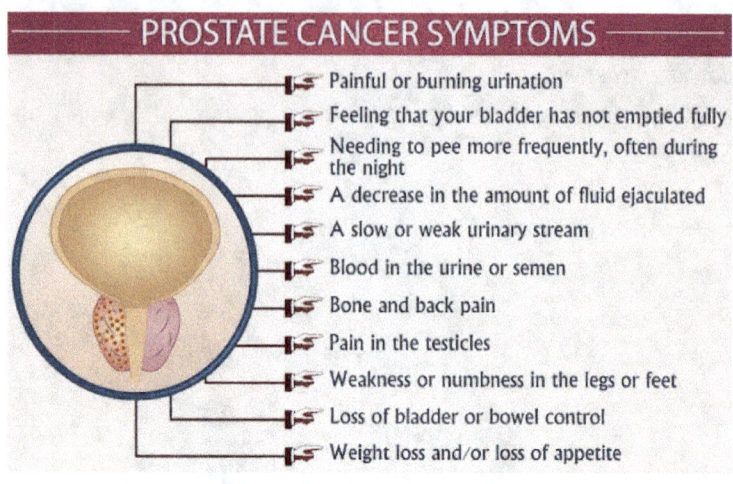

*Family, this picture shows the known
early warning signs of prostate problems. The key is to go and
notify your doctor. Remember, early detection is the best prevention.* [7]

---

[7] Image credit: Shutterstock.com

3

Shaw's Victory over Cancer

This layer of cancer's definition, simplified, is when diseased cells divide uncontrollably, and spread to surrounding tissues in the body, altering our DNA or genes.

First things first: cancer is cancer. There are many forms, and it is the second leading cause of human death in the United States, according to 2024 data (American Cancer Statistics). In the African American race, there are socioeconomic factors that put Black people at higher risk, and twice as likely to die. Some of those factors are lack of proper insurance, diets, and lifestyles that increase the risk of diseases.

In our family, we did not have medical insurance

consistently because of the type of jobs my parents had to accept. My mom worked for people who paid cash back then and didn't offer insurance during the sixties. My dad did have insurance, but at that time, cancer was still a bit of a mystery disease that a lot of people didn't understand.

Family, it was basically about survival, and we relied on the Food and Drug Administration to protect our race. I know my family did not have any clue about cancer, and health checks were for the basics like heart checks, dental, or pregnancy for women.

The leading causes of death for African Americans are heart diseases and cancers. Knowing your health digits is an essential part of managing your overall health and living well.

"Let's go," Family! Go where?

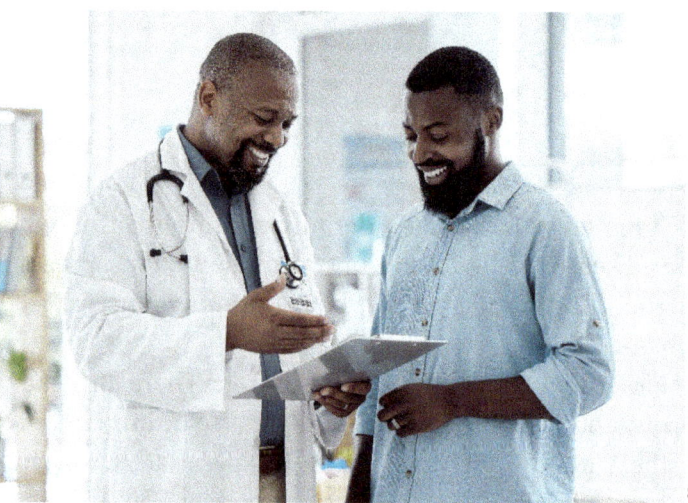

Get your health check-up!

In 1998, at the age of forty-four, my oldest brother, James, was diagnosed with a rare form of stomach cancer.

---

[8] Image credit: iStock by Getty Images

He was a United States Marine assigned to Camp Lejeune, North Carolina. He was stationed there from 1972 through 1975, and was impacted by the water contamination mixed with cleaning agents. James passed away due to stomach cancer in 2000, eighteen years after the incident at Camp Lejune, which became public knowledge in 1982.

I was ten years younger, at age thirty-four. The impact of knowing he did not catch it early, drove me to get tested at my annual physical with both DRE and PSA blood tests.

I was determined to use family history to ensure that my brothers and I were focused and not blindsided by this disease. It's personal, and I became determined to fight like a warrior to beat back cancer from attacking our family.

Shaw's Family History Journal

Name and Birth Order	Age Diagnosed	Comments
James	44	Died at age 46
*Sibling	61	6 months free
Darnell	50	11 years free
*Sibling	47	13 years free

Individuals who would like to remain anonymous.

At the time of writing this book, my next older brother, at age sixty-one, was diagnosed and is currently being treated for prostate cancer. What I like most about my brother's cancer journey is his faith! I can remember his words, "the good Lord's Will be done, and I'm ok with the outcome!" For me, that shows strong faith that no matter the outcome it's well with his Spirit.

He is going through proton therapy, which has a high success rate, and patients rave about not having surgery and having little side effects. Family, proton therapy, or proton beam, delivers a pinpointed beam of radiation to destroy your cancer cells at a precise tumor location. This works great to minimize damage to healthy tissues around the tumor.

The rate for being cancer-free is based on risk and early detection!

- 99% low risk
- 94% medium risk
- 74% high risk[9]

A choice I wish I had considered years earlier. It would be a game changer for me, in hindsight.

An update on my older brother; after proton treatment, he is cancer-free and living well with little to no major side effects!

In the spring of 2011, my youngest brother, at age forty-seven, found out during his routine health exams—the DRE and PSA results—would later be a cancer diagnosis. After learning the news, he chose to have his prostate removed and focused on living!

This news floored me—wondering how this could be. The cancer had skipped two brothers and attacked the oldest and youngest siblings. *Wow, it's personal,* and we

---

[9] Data credit: National Library of Medicine
https://www.ncbi.nlm.nih.gov/pmc/articles/PMC5705018/

started questioning how this could be. Was it food, or where we lived? Did burning fossil fuels, black coal, or wood-burning stoves cause it?

We will never know!

My older brother and I were perplexed, so we supported my younger brother with encouragement and emotional support.

My younger brother used his mancave, a small ten feet wide by eleven feet long gazebo that was enclosed and finished inside. We had dedicated it as a place to honor God and relax and discuss men-related topics and pride-related topics that men can share with one another, code stuff that stays close to our hearts! We made it comfortable with lawn chairs, a table, television, fans in summer, heat in the winter. This was his secret worship place, as he would always have his Bible open, and for me, this was epic for his faith, as he was putting his actions to work by actively searching for understanding and knowledge. He walked the talk, and he was healed from cancer! As brothers, some of our discussions were about the following:

- Healing from inside out without straining
- Urinary incontinence and bladder self-control
- Erectile dysfunction, and getting back in the game
- Lifestyle shifts, such as no more kids, wife's impact without sex during healing period
- Sexual needs after the healing period, pill, etc.
- Spiritual needs, mental and emotional impact

Family, these are topics all men need to know when having this type of diagnosis. Recovering from surgery is a lengthy process that requires time and patience and lots of endurance plus family support and coaching from friends too.

Confess and believe and do what my brother and I did. Confessing to God's words unlocks His promises as recorded in the Bible. Life for my younger brother after an eight-week recovery period returned to a place where he could do his normal routine. His recovery went extremely well with little to no major issues, and he's living his best life. Good health is wealth and by going to the doctor, he lived to see another day, birthday, anniversary, and his son's graduation from high school. For him, his main advantage was to be cancer-free and live a full life with his family. *"Let's Go!"*

Back to me, Family, let's fast forward the years as I was diligent about my prostate exams (DRE/PSA) and tracking my digits. At the ripe age of fifty, during my semi-annual health check, I was informed by my doctor that my PSA had gone up two-plus points. He also said that there could be something going on inside the prostate and that a biopsy would show what was happening. I said, "Biopsy, what's that?"

He informed me that it is a short procedure to look at the prostate, where you're given general anesthesia for mild pain, as they go into the anus with a scope. Then, specialized instruments work side-by-side with the doctors' eyes, looking through the scope and collecting samples from different areas of the prostate.

I know what you're thinking, Family, *"Wow! That sounds painful." Well, let's say, it's not that bad and you can get some light pain medication to ease the feelings during the procedure and afterward.*

Even knowing this, it was wild to think they were going to take multiple samples of my prostate. Family, I remember hoping I wouldn't feel anything, and of course, wouldn't bleed.

By the time I left, he gave me a clear assurance that I would be okay, and a handful of pamphlets about the biopsy procedure.

That night, after hearing that I had the potential of prostate cancer, I thought to myself, *please, don't let that be true*. And if it was true—hopefully I had caught it early enough to treat or remove it.

Let me tell you, there was a feeling in the pit of my belly that said, *"I got you. All sickness is not unto death according to the Word of God."*

Yes, oh yes, I parked my faith in this promise, believed it, and took my tail to sleep!

The next day, I called my younger brother, who beat this disease through prayer and believing God's Word, which said, "By your stripes, I am healed." The power of words matters as we have what we say as stated in the Bible. The Book of Genesis chapter 1:3 says, "Then God said, 'Let there be light,' and there was light."

We also know that healing is the children of God's bread.

Knowing this promise of God, we park our belief and faith on what we know, and it is so! Next, we have healing and the power to receive what we believe. I speak and declare that whosoever is reading this book can be assured, every promise of God is true to those who accept him by faith. To accept him, you must confess with your mouth that Jesus Christ is your Lord and Savior, and he paid the ultimate price of dying for your sins and rose on the third day with all power.

All you must do is confess to get connected to the Kingdom of God in your local community. So, Family, see how powerful words are to you in living a powerful life of health and healing.

Our God, Jehovah, can be whatever you need him to be. Jehovah-Rapha healer is what he is to me.

For me, Family, I created a prayer closet or praying war room in my home upstairs in one of my spare bedrooms. I took everything out of the closet and put my Army battle dress uniform or military clothing on hangers and hung them there for war against negative thoughts.

I put my bible in there and use the space as my secret closet to tap into my spirit man and align the mind and body and soul. The size of the closet was only three and one-half feet wide and about five feet long, so being five-feet eleven-inches tall I could barely sit and not even lay down, but it was perfect for kneeling. It would be fine with me if I could get on my knees to pray. For comfort I took a thick queen-size mattress pad and doubled-folded it to pad the floor and close the door. My objective was to cut out the lights and not see any light under the bottom of the door. I took the back wall in the walk-in closet and put positive messages and scriptures of healing and reminded myself that I can do all things through my savior, Jesus Christ. The battle of the mind is where we must fight the fiery dart of the enemy. Being in the dark closet helped, it is like having your eyes closed at night. This took away my sight and caused my sense of sight to shift internally to visions of what healing and walking on the other side of being cancer-free looks like. In the Bible, the book of Luke chapter 8:40 talks about how Jesus heals us according to our faith. In this chapter, I used the example of a local leader of the synagogue Jairus, Luke 8:41, who exercised great faith when his daughter was sick, and Jesus healed her when the crowd said she was dead. Jesus told the crowd to leave, and that the girl was asleep and they laughed at him. "Then Jesus took her by the hand and said in a loud voice, 'My child, get up!' And at that moment her life returned, and she immediately stood up!" (Luke 8:54–55). Examples like this helped me stay strong. Then I was reminded while that was going on, a woman with an issue of blood saw Jesus and reached through the crowd and touched his gown and was healed.

My prayer closet actions carried me through seen and unseen energy shifts, both highs and lows that brought on tears and pain at times. Through the trials of healing, I stood on my faith and did not let go of it. At times, I could see darkness and laying for twenty to forty minutes or so things changed, and I could see mental pictures of images like negative photos in a dark room that was as real as a slow-motion picture movie. It would come in and out as I processed my spiritual healing journey. This became a nightly process for me and other times I would just drift off to sleep and drift back in and stay disciplined in my routine.

For nine months, I stayed true to doing this and with my family's support in prayer I knew that it was only time before the manifestation would take place in my life. Family, Jesus is my provider, Jehovah-Jireh is my God. He takes care of all my needs. He is my Abba or Father, my source! Always on time!

Family, I have all the confidence knowing that my brother's God is my God too! The Brother's Keeper promises God is true to his Word, and I believe it one hundred percent. My God keeps all his promises. You see a promise keeper is committed to practicing spiritual, ethical, moral, and sexual purity. We must practice what is preached. When we do this, our marriages and relationships become stronger, and our families are blessed and protected.

Our belief in God's Word matters and we inherit all the promises of the Kingdom of God.

As I prepared for the biopsy, it was time to decide, but I knew that I was healed before this procedure even began. Family and faith require you to see it before you experience it! This is the only way to bring it to pass!

The biopsy proceeded, and the pain was not too bad; I only felt a slight pinch here and there, and before I knew it, the medical technician said, "Mr. Shaw, we are done."

I replied aloud, "Wow, that was only fifteen minutes, yes, sir!"

"The next step is for us to take your samples to the lab, have them tested, and proceed from there, which takes about two weeks."

Now comes the testing of faith; yes, talk about faith. This was a trying time when the enemy, the devil, tried to put thoughts, ideas, and suggestions in my mind to cause havoc.

Family, I said, *"Oh no!"*

After taking hold of my Bible, the Word of God, I stood firm on what I believed and knew—that all things would work out for my good. The next seven days went by, and I received an early message from my doctor on December twenty-third that my results were positive. He said I had multiple areas with cancer on the prostate. Man, I told him I wanted to see the results and upon looking at the numbers, it was true and difficult to swallow.

So, I went home to my war room, got on my knees, and began to pray, asking God for direction. After breathing deeply and pausing, I knew that everything would be okay.

Later that day, I shared my results with my mother, who told me everything would be all right. I believed her and was glad I had her support and confidence.

When you have major life-altering news, it's not good to let pride cause you to keep secrets.

It seems that as a Black man we are taught to not show any weakness in public, and this was one disease that put you in crisis mode real fast, this is as real as it gets. You don't want others in your personal business at all. Let me tell you, pride will knock you way down if you let it, Family.

What I recommend is to let go and let family and friends in as soon as possible to assist you with getting the best help possible to live well and see another phase of life!

The key to healing is to trust and let your faith work by letting a few prayer warriors in to work on your behalf. The power of prayer works, Family, and gives you hope to sustain you in the anticipation of signs, wonders, or miracles.

My decision came quickly through the Holy Spirit in a revelation download on Christmas Eve. The Holy Spirit instructed me to have my prostate removed as quickly as possible. I was to have it done at a veteran hospital with the best surgeon, *my angel*, Dr. B. J., a regional expert in robotic prostatectomy surgery at the veteran's hospital. My blessed assurance was knowing this was my younger brother's choice that he made two and half years ago and he had healed and recovered just fine.

As time would have it, during the Christmas holidays, I shared my cancer diagnosis with my immediate family and closest friends. Just talking to them helped me cope with thoughts that kept coming into my mind. The overwhelming support and prayers carried me through the holidays. I realized that this was a test of my faith and that the best way to overcome cancer is to go through the process head-on. At night, when I was all alone, it seemed the worst. Thoughts kept popping up about cancer destroying my body, so removing the prostate would surely prevent that from happening. My next major hurdle was when I could get this done. Followed by how long the procedure will take to recover or heal. Stay with me, and *let's go* see what the end will be! My belief and faith are "I am a conqueror!" Jehovah-Ralpha healer!

4

Cancer Diagnosis and Treatment Options

In early January 2014, I had several follow-up appointments at the veteran hospital. My urologist noted that I was in good shape and my overall health was excellent. He suggested that I would be able to get on the list for surgery right away. This was all I needed to hear, and it was what my spiritual download showed me on Christmas Eve in December.

The following week, I got a call that my procedure was scheduled for April 1, 2014, and I would be contacted by the surgery staff with details on the pre-operative instructions.

The first thought was—*it's on and popping.* Cancer is about to be a thing of the past. I made up my mind that

I was going to get into the best shape of my life, so my healing from the procedure and recovery would be minimized. I also started to read more about what to eat and what to avoid, like fried foods and high-fat foods. My Faith went into action, and my mind was made up that I was a winner. All my thoughts and beliefs reassured me that I had what it takes to beat this one hundred percent. Having a computer helped me research what causes cancer and what races are more susceptible to having cancer.

Go figure, Black men are at the highest risk, and statistics show we are 70 percent more likely to develop prostate cancer. Guess what else I found out, Family? We are twice as likely to die from this disease. One of the major things we as men are so prideful and try and keep secrets until it is too late. We are less likely to go get a yearly health checkup.

Here is what I experienced over the last ten years: men I personally knew, or knew *of*, in positions of power from Civil Rights leaders, news broadcasters, military leaders, mayors, movie stars, NFL and NBA players, to Kingdom Men, have been diagnosed with prostate cancer. My point is cancer does not discriminate and it's up to us men to start talking and keeping this in front of all men regardless of age, race, or skin color. *"Let's Go!"* Go where? Get our wealth which is health.

. . .

There are many options to get rid of prostate cancer and I would like to explore some of what I know as being cutting-edge. Here is a list of ten options that I wanted to share and does not represent everything that's out.

- Hormone Therapy
- Proton Beam Radiation Therapy
- Radical Laparoscopic Prostatectomy
- Open Radical Prostatectomy
- Chemotherapy
- Radiation Treatment
- Targeted Therapy
- Laser Therapy
- Immunotherapy
- High Intensity Ultrasound

The list above is only intended to get you thinking about how curable prostate cancer can be. Let's consider this option first, if you catch it early through getting a health check DRE or PSA, or both, you can win the battle. Family, *"Let's go!"* Your health is your wealth!

I am neither a doctor nor make claims to discuss any of the above options except what I experienced. My choice was to have an Open Radical Laparoscopic Prostatectomy done as soon as possible on April 1, 2014. So, I prepared and got ready by having my family present, and on the day before my surgery, I got a call saying it was canceled due to an emergency procedure.

Talk about April Fools', I was quite disappointed and just took it as a sign that God has a reason for everything. Family, I had gotten ready with my siblings and Mom, traveling four hours, only to get rejected on the first of April. My mental state and emotional health shifted at first, then I took advantage of the visit to enjoy their presence. On the third of April, I got rescheduled to the end of the month on the twenty-eighth of April at 11:00 a.m.

The morning of my procedure, I arrived early, around 7:00 a.m., to do my pre-operative checks and get all scrubbed, checked, and wired for show time at 11:00 a.m. sharp. My surgeon, Dr. B. J. came in and talked to me and asked what procedure I was having done, plus to confirm I was in the right state of mind before he performed the surgery.

His next question was what my name was, so he was sure to operate on the right person. After confirming that I was the right patient, he put his initials on my stomach to confirm the exact area and to let the team know he was sure he had the right patient.

So, as soon as he left, here came the anesthesiologist who asked about the prior surgeries and if I was allergic to any medication, and I told them I was not. He said he was going to use propofol to put me to sleep, and he would be monitoring me the whole time. *Wow, this is great,* I thought. I was very pleased with the level of care, and just took a deep breath!

The next thing I knew was that the doctor inserted the medication into my veins. And, Family, I was out like a light.

Dr. B. J. performed an Open Radical Laparoscopic Prostatectomy on my abdomen area with five small incisions. There was also another smaller incision on my lower left side to drain fluid.

So, Dr. B. J's team worked on my body with five open tubes inserted with cameras or other medical instruments. The procedure also used carbon gas to inflate my abdomen. It allowed visibility for the optical scopes.

Then he used the scopes as guides and worked on the computer using high-tech paddles like joy sticks, guiding the instruments for the removal process.

That is all I knew from talking to him before and after my procedure. The procedure lasted about three and a half hours, and I was told I had only lost half a pint of blood. He buttoned my abdomen up with self-dissolving stitches, took my prostate and two seminal vesicles out, and sent it to the laboratory for testing. Please note, that was the end of sperm production for me, as my hardware was clipped and stopped sperm seed reproduction.

Next came the post-operative process where I woke up in a bit of pain in my belly and scrotum area that on a scale of one to ten peaked at nine.

Yes, Family, I was on fire and had a sharp piercing pain shooting deep inside my testicles. All I knew was I needed some pain pills and plenty of ice. The ice packs were my new best friend as I couldn't keep enough of them around my testicle and lower belly. Next was the catheter (tube) inserted in my penis head connected to my bladder to drain the urine. This was sore too. Later, about three or four hours post-operation, the pain became manageable, and it was time to get up and start walking to show that I was ready to go home in twenty-four to forty-eight hours.

My objective before the procedure was to only spend twenty-four hours in the hospital and get moving to the other side of healing.

That evening, about five hours after the procedure, I got up with the nurse's assistance. My anxiety kicked in once I got back into my room.

Family, I am telling you—that had to be the smallest hospital room I have ever been in! Upon complaining to the charge nurse, I was upgraded to a hospital suite that felt like a hotel room with all the bells and whistles.

Talk about the favor of God. It opened up on me that evening, and I was truly taken care of well at the veteran hospital. The medical team was first-class and made my experience as pleasant as possible.

I walked about every two hours to manage the pain and to keep my anxiety down. As I passed the nurse's workstation, they said, "Sir, you're doing as well, as I did three laps every two hours." At about four in the morning, I was walking and wanted to get off the floor, so I asked if I could go downstairs. The next thing I knew, I was in the doorway, and it opened. *Wow, it felt oh so, so good!* The next thing I knew was I walked out about two feet and stopped to truly get maximum air in my lungs to calm my anxiety.

The doors closed and I stood there for two minutes with my medical stand and holding my hospital gown that was half open in the rear. My tail got cold quickly, so I met my objective of getting some fresh air and relaxing for one hundred and twenty seconds. It felt so good to breathe the night air.

I turned around to walk two steps back into the main door. To my surprise, the door would not open and I panicked, then went into flight or fight mode and said to myself, *"Ranger, it's time to think on your feet!"* So, I came up with a plan to go to the emergency room entrance and take my tail back upstairs!

The plan worked with no issues. I got back upstairs and took a small nap, and before I knew it, the nurses were making their last rounds before shift change. My pain got better, and by seven in the morning, I had my pain down to level five or six.

The next morning, the physician assistant came in and looked at how well I was doing. The assistant said that I could be discharged after lunch!

They didn't have to tell me twice! I got into prep mode and packed my personal items and went straight home with family.

Next was my follow-up appointment to see how things

were healing and take my catheter out of my bladder though using a tube in my penis. Talk about awkward things, it worked fine as I managed for seven days. One thing I wanted to point out is that ice packs became my best friend as I put them on the testicles every few hours to keep the swelling down. As time went on the pain decreased and I felt so relieved that God answered my prayers and spared my life!

My prostate and two seminal vesicles went to the lab and came back, positive for prostate cancer. The disease was contained in the prostate site. After a biopsy, there is a score given called a Gleason score which shows how likely or aggressive the cancer cells may spread. The range is from one to ten and the lower the better. My Gleason score was seven on both sides and all the disease was inside with no contact with any other part of my body. Early detection is key to survival and quick intervention! *"Let's Go," Family!*

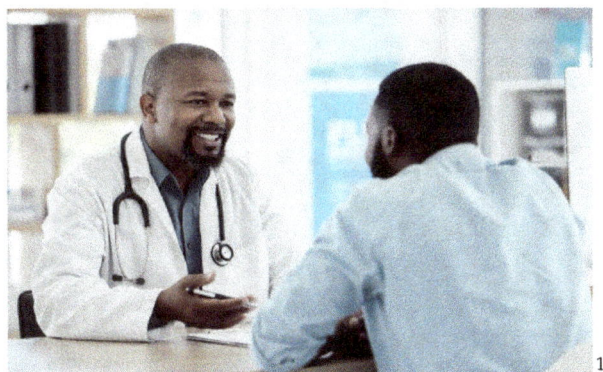

The best resource is your healthcare provider for expert care and guidance for your needs.

---

[10] Image credit: iStock by Getty Images

My mission now is to educate all men on their choices so they can reduce the risk of erectile dysfunction and loss of reproduction. You got this, man!

5

Erectile Dysfunction and Mental Struggles

After an Open Radical Prostatectomy, there are going to be some major adjustments that will have to be understood before you choose your medical option. Let's explore erectile dysfunction, a symptom that most men will experience after surgical treatment.

Erectile dysfunction (ED) is the inability to get and hold a hard erection during sexual intercourse. There are many reasons for ED issues, and I will attempt to discuss a few things to get you thinking about what to expect after surgery. Please note, I am not a doctor, and my opinions only reflect what my life experiences have taught me and talking to my doctor. Your best source of information for ED is your doctor, as we are all different.

So, *let's go!*

Erectile dysfunction is caused by so many factors and can be corrected with the right treatments. Health is wealth and ED is a breakdown in your sexual health.

One of the major things I want to point out is that ED can influence self-esteem and can create tension in relationships.

Sexual intimacy is very important and affects both men and women's behaviors differently when ED interrupts the flow of sexual intercourse. Let's explore some known issues.

Erectile dysfunction's common cause is:

- Treatment for Prostate Cancer
- Heart Disease
- Diabetes
- Overweight and Obesity
- Sleep disorders
- Alcoholism and substance abuse
- Smoking
- Certain prescription medications
- High Blood Pressure or Cholesterol
- Enlarge Prostate

Now that I have pointed out that there are many reasons for ED. Let me share my journey of Prostate Cancer and be as transparent as possible as I battled erectile dysfunction. Before the procedure I had no issues with ED and my sexual life was normal and very satisfying up to age fifty-one.

I had been married and had two healthy children who are grown and started lives of their own. Since then, I divorced and had already fulfilled my purpose of being a Kingdom Man by producing two lovely children.

Remember, Family, no prostate and seminal gland equals no sperm to create life.

This is key to know and understand when choosing to have the prostate removed at an early age.

First, let's look at the mental health struggles I faced after the Radical Prostatectomy operation. The main obstacle was how to accept that I went from having a healthy sex life to dealing with erectile dysfunction in the prime of life.

As a man, this is huge, and having no control of your penis movement and natural brain signal puts you in a state of depression. Did you know that it's normal for the average man to have ten or more erections per day and three to five at night while sleeping? The next obstacle is urinary incontinence, which is having poor bladder control. This happened to me right after surgery and it was so embarrassing. It made me very upset, to the point I wanted to stay home. My urologist prescribed men's incontinence liners to help with this.

At first, I refused to use them. It wasn't until I put my pride aside that I actually tried it. This small adjustment gave me more confidence to get going on the road to recovery.

After several months and working on staying physically active, things improved mentally, and I started looking at steps to work toward removing erectile dysfunction.

What bothered me was when I was doing work or bending down, I leaked into my underwear. This feeling took me into a place and space mentally that deterred me from interacting with females who were not a part of my immediate family.

Seven months went by before I had the confidence to try some of the recommended devices for ED. Let's explore some of the devices that were recommended to me by my urologist team to assist with gaining and maintaining an erection. The first thing I did was work on rebuilding my muscle controls post-surgery performing Kegel exercises.

These exercises work the pelvic floor by squeezing your butt and tightening your lower stomach to work the muscles for bladder control. The physical therapy team will guide you through the science behind the movement to strengthen and get you back in shape.

Here are some of the devices to consider for erectile dysfunction. I have firsthand experiences with several of the devices below so let's explore some of these. I chose to use a progressive approach to solve my ED problem.

- Natural remedies
- Prescription Pills
- Vacuum pumps and holding rings
- Penile injection
- Urethral suppositories
- Penile implant(s) (BINGO!!!)
- Topical Gels and creams

Family, let us win by opening up to allow our healthcare providers to guide you through your individual needs that's tailored to your diagnosis and recovery.

A vacuum device, as shown on the next page, draws and creates an erection by pulling blood into the penis. This a good way to get blood circulation into the penis and to hold it there you may require an elastic ring at the base as shown on the next page.

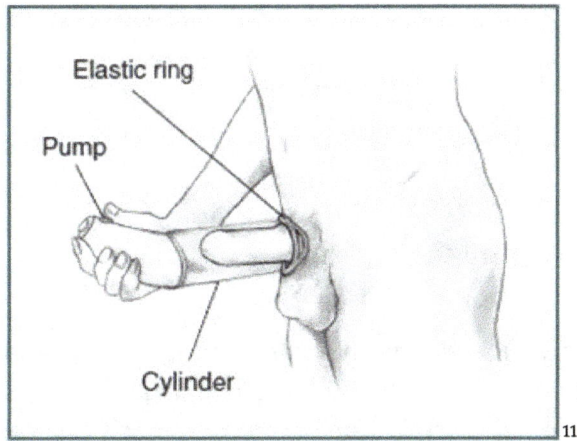

AMS 700™ Inflatable Penile Implant

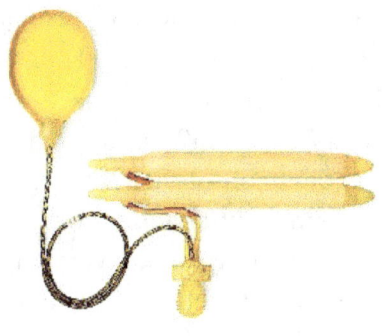

---

[11] Image credit: National Institute of Diabetes and Digestive and Kidney Diseases (NIDDK), part of the National Institutes of Health.
[12] Image provided courtesy of Boston Scientific. ©2024 Boston Scientific Corporation or its affiliates. All rights reserved.
https://www.bostonscientific.com/en-US/education.html

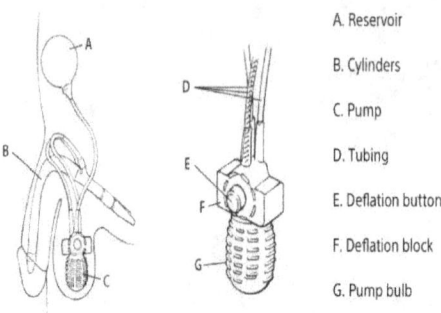

A. Reservoir
B. Cylinders
C. Pump
D. Tubing
E. Deflation button
F. Deflation block
G. Pump bulb
[13]

This device was my choice to eliminate ED for good and solve the mental and emotional health challenges of sexual intimacy. The success rate of this system is 95 percent patient satisfaction, which worked well for me. My BINGO! It was a game-changer for my ED issues. Let me say this to all who are reading and learning about ED.

It's a step-by-step process, so my best advice is seeking wisdom from your doctor. Family, here is where you need support alongside you for the journey back to full sexual health. Please, I'll say it twice—don't let pride get in the way of your recovery, and you'll return to normalcy more quickly. There are plenty of self-help videos on penile implants from semi-rigid to inflatable devices by searching on the internet. I landed here and am very happy with not having any more issues with erectile dysfunction.

Let's Go! Health is Wealth. Love yourself and live well, Kingdom Man, you have the victory!

---

[13] AMS 700 TM with Inflatable Penile Prosthesis is intended for use in the treatment of male erectile dysfunction (impotence). Implanting a penile prosthesis will damage or destroy any remaining ability to have a natural erection, as well as make other treatment options (oral medications, vacuum devices, or injections) impossible. All images are the property of Boston Scientific. All trademarks are the property of their respective owners.

6

Intimacy and Sex

Let's peel back the layers and talk about sex and intimacy after prostate cancer. One of the things that I experienced is when you take sex out of a man's life, it creates the strangest feeling of not being whole or manly. Your confidence is shaken as you re-adjust to who you are now. This was my personal experience as well as talking to some close friends battling the disease. All during the preoperative and post recovery I lost all interest in sex but not the intimacy with my partner. What I learned and focused on was that we were *designed* to be in a relationship with one another.

Our physical touching is key to communication before, during, and after sexual intimacy. My partner walked through the journey and embraced me with love and kindness as she understood that intimacy and sex required healing and patience.

There are five love languages that you may be familiar with that Baptist Minister Dr. Gary Chapman speaks of in his book, *The 5 Love Languages.*

It's written to show you how to understand and recognize differences and gives you the tools to express a heartfelt commitment to your mate. The book was first published in 1992. It helped me by outlining general ways that romantic partners express and experience love. He calls them "love languages." I studied these and committed them to memory, found out my primary and secondary love languages, and shared them with my partner so there was no "guessing" how to please me. The five love languages are:

1. Quality Time
2. Acts of Service
3. Physical Touch
4. Words of Affirmation
5. Receiving Gifts

There is a short love language survey you can take and identify your love languages in order of importance to your individual needs.

Read *The 5 Love Languages* by Gary Chapman to learn more about them.

In my relationship, *quality time* and *physical touch* were the most important ways I felt loved by my partner.

Finally, the healing from erectile dysfunction was over and I had a new way to enjoy sexual intercourse with confidence. My life blossomed with the penile implant as I was able to have an erection for 5, 10, 15, 20, 25, 30 or more minutes. It works, and is a game changer, and I love the way it's private plus transparent to my sex partner. The intercourse feeling was different for me at first, but the results were still the same and *very pleasing*. I call this sexual intimacy the "new normal" without seminal glands or vesicles to produce sperm. That's right, no sperm without the prostate, and its jewels the seminal glands. The penis still goes through the normal orgasm feelings and my quality of life significantly improved.

My health became wealthy again as I navigated through sexual intimacy and knew how to manage my feelings and abilities during sex. My self-esteem peaked knowing that I had full control of my erections and no more ED issues.

In July of 2020, the greatest thing happened to me. I got into a new relationship and got married in November of 2021. My life changed, and the new normal was a thing of the past. I have learned what techniques work best sexually and intimately for me and my wife that far exceeds my wildest imagination of pleasure.

Sexual intimacy in a new marriage is a couple's priority, like a beautiful sunflower that grows upward when you feed and nourish it properly. I like to say, "The sky is the limit when you love someone." I have eight years of experience, and I am glad I made this choice to get the penile implant for erectile dysfunction.

My experience with the AMS 700™ Inflatable Penile Implant has been a game changer after cancer tried to shut down my sexual pleasures.

It takes some time to learn the device. The learning curve is simple once you get the basic steps of penile inflation and release.

The cool thing about the implant is that it's undetectable and installed in the lower parts of your penis and scrotums with no exposed parts. The average woman would never know you have an implant unless you shared the details.

To the man on the fence, do consider all your options, and know that there is sexual help and a fun life after an erectile dysfunction diagnosis. I am a witness and just say to all of you, "Go! Go!"

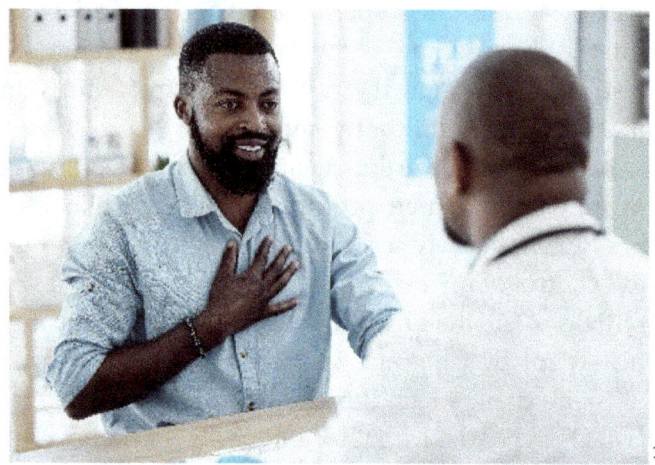

Family, the picture above shows heartfelt lines of communication between yourself and a healthcare professional. Be honest about your health by going to the experts to find what works best for you.

---

[14] Image credit: iStock by Getty Image

7

Physical Touch Post-Surgery Q&A

The last layer is physical touch. Daily stimulation is so important to staying healthy when you're battling erectile dysfunction. The muscles and blood vessels in the penis need to be stimulated to stay healthy and responsive. Remember my earlier comment that a normal man has about ten erections a day, and three or more while sleeping at night?

Daily use of the implant is a critical management practice that keeps your penis muscles healthy and flexible for game day! For a healthy sex life, a key point I want to stress, alert, or inform, is that a change in your brain signal may happen. However, you need to know that it may require time to get things moving again like before. Remember nerves have to grow back for tissue that has been cut.

This can be performed while bathing or in bed, just have a routine that works for you.

The post-surgery visit with your urologist will send you on your way to go experiment with your sex partner.

Effective communication is critical, so your sex partner is aware of the changes that have occurred within your body. It is always a good practice to be upfront and have your sex partner know in advance that you're recovering from prostate cancer and erectile dysfunction. In the long run, it will serve you best to be as transparent as possible about any health-related issues. This practice goes both ways. Let me be real and tell you no two men's recovery will be the same. Our bodies and DNA are unique, and you and your doctor are the experts so talk and hold your doctor accountable for your details. Nerve spearing is key to minimizing erectile dysfunction during surgery and removal of the prostate. When a nerve is impacted it takes some time to grow and respond and therapy is needed. Men, it's important to understand this before getting diagnosed so you can take the minimum evasive surgery approach.

Proton therapy or beam therapy has been around for some time and many men choose this option based on early detection.

You and your doctor are the experts so explore all your options and do not rush to choose.

Mentally, it's weighty on the mind so know it's a slow growth and your urology doctor is the expert. Health is wealth! *"Let's Go!"* Go get that prostate checked! *As an African American with four out of four brothers having cancer, I highly recommend getting checked as soon as possible.* There is a standard based on American Cancer Society data, however, Blacks are at higher risk. I am pushing for the DRE test and PSA test to start at the age of thirty-five to have a good baseline of your digits.

Early detection is a key factor in a minimum evasive approach to fighting a cancer diagnosis. I have created some questions and answers to get you thinking about what questions to ask your doctor.

The following items are wellness resources: Prostate Health Card, Prostate Health Recorder, and Family Medical History Recorder to track and monitor your prostate results.

The cards were developed to carry and remind you of PSA and DRE digits, which are must-haves for monitoring your health over time. It's your gift to yourself or your loved ones to take control of your body to live well. A few journal pages are also included to keep things in one place.

Questions and Answers

1. How do cancer diagnoses affect emotions?

    Answer: Family, cancer affects your physical health and it's normal to expect it to bring up a wide range of emotions as well. We can experience a wide range of emotions like sadness, fear, anger, stress, disgust, and anxiety. These feelings are normal, and to be expected. This can affect you and your family.

2. What are some coping methods to deal with spikes in emotions for you and your family?

    Answer: Let me say this to you, Family, there is no wrong way, it depends on your faith and beliefs. What helps is to educate yourself and learn about your specific situation. This can give you some control over your choices of treatment. For some, it may shift to doing other things, hobbies, crafts to distract attention away from cancer.

3. How long does it take to recover from prostate cancer?

Answer: It depends on how early the cancer is detected and what stage you find out you have the diagnosis. For example, the surgery recovery time is normally six to eight weeks and longer for advanced stages of cancer. Early testing and annual physicals help to reduce risk and recovery time from cancer.

4. What is the best method to detect cancer in Black men?

Answer: There are methods to detect prostate cancer, one is the Digital Rectal Examination and Prostate Specific Antigen blood test. It's a good idea to start early if you have a family history. Let your doctor guide you and take control. I am recommending age thirty-five for high-risk families.

5. Why is family history so important?

Answer: Family history gives you advanced indicators as to what genetic health issues affect your family. If you don't have data, ask relatives about your family tree. Be a change agent. Record yours and pass it to your offspring.

6. At what age should I have my prostate examined?

Answer: It depends on family history as to whether cancer runs in your family. The average age is forty to fifty. Sooner for Black men, who are at greater risk. Recommend age thirty-five, for family history.

7. What are the signs I have prostate issues and should have it looked at?

   Answer: First, you should always check with your doctor for any issues with your penis, bladder, or prostate. Slow streams, bleeding, having to urinate multiple times throughout the night, and issues with erectile dysfunction. Your doctor is an expert. Go get checked for a piece of mind and use your benefits!

8. When is a prostate biopsy needed?

   Answer: A biopsy is a minor procedure to collect samples from the prostate. The procedure takes about fifteen minutes. The doctor will order a biopsy if they see an increase in your PSA or feel something swollen during a DRE examination.

9. Can prostate cancer be cured?

   Answer: **Prostate cancer can be cured. Yes, it can.** Ask your doctor for the best method for your specific situation. Early testing is a key factor in this silent disease. The good news is that the prostate cancer survival rate is 97.5 percent and improving with advances in technology. The American Cancer Society reports 97 percent or higher with a five-year success rate based on the stage the cancer is detected. *Just Go!*

10. How do diet and exercise affect your chances of getting prostate cancer?

    Answer: It is always a good idea to eat healthily and exercise. This will allow your immune system to work more efficiently to resist diseases. Seek your doctor's advice before making changes to your diet or wellness routine.

11. Is prostate cancer contagious?

    Answer: Cancer is not contagious. You cannot catch cancer from someone else. There is no risk with sexual activity.

12. How long can I live with prostate cancer?

    Answer: That is for doctors and the good Lord to answer. See, medical advice miracles happen every day. Just go to your doctor.

13. How do the underprivileged maintain hope during this cancer medical journey?

    Answer: Family, once you accept or reject the illness, get you a routine that gives you a sense of new hope and purpose for living. Remember, others have traveled this road and live to share their story. You got this, Family!

    There is help on the horizon for Medicare beneficiaries through the following FIND ACT of 2023. Facilitating Innovative Nuclear Diagnostics (FIND) Act of 2023 (S. 1544/H.R. 1199) to assist with cost and care. Congress, we need to push this through!

    Consider dedicating your time to helping others and see your prayers and blessings come back to you! *"Just go!"*

14. What if I don't have any family nearby or live alone?

    Answer: Let me suggest you reach out to your local cancer support groups. Most doctors or social workers can assist you with a list. Here are some online resources:

- National Cancer Institute: www.cancer.gov/about-cancer/coping/adjusting-to-cancer/support-groups
- The Prostate Health Education Network (PHEN): https://www.prostatehealthed.org/ PHEN can assist with providing guidance to African American men and help with disparity solutions steering you through your journey.

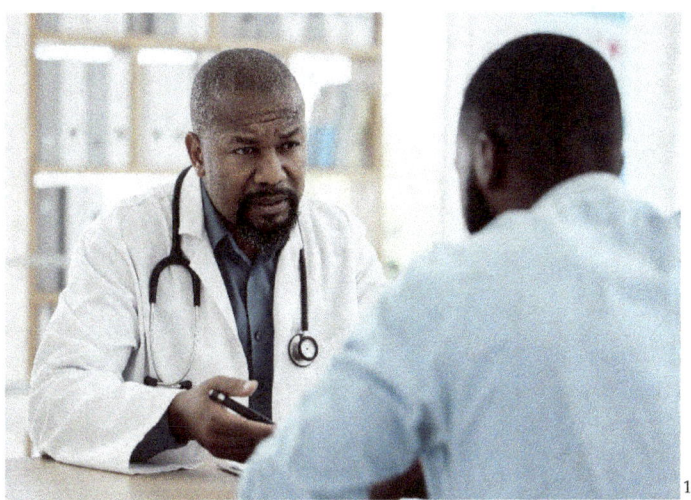

Family, you're not in this alone. Allow cancer support groups to give you encouragement and resources to cope with your specific situation.

---

[15] Image credit: iStock by Getty Images

Acknowledgments

My journey in life has not been easy. However, it's been a good route of travel with little to no regrets. When I think things over and look at what has occurred, I give all the Glory to Abba, my Father in Heaven, who loads me with daily benefits. Jesus is the reason for my success, and I am winning in life with His favor. If you don't know Him, I highly suggest you get to know Jesus Christ, my Lord and Savior.

True story: on July 26, 2023, I had back surgery level two, where the doctor replaced two lumbar joints (L2-L5) and fused them with two Titanium spacers and three Titanium rods. I still have reasonable mobility and always strive to be positive because there is always someone worse off. Eleven years of cancer-free diagnosis—truly a blessing.

"I walk by faith, not by sight," is my motto. Thank you for taking the time to read my story. It's my *hope* you are sharpened by the transparency of what men need to know.

If you're that man, this is for you, and walk through my journey to let go of pride, and sharpen another man! I want to thank all those who have poured into my life: God, Mom, brothers, sisters, friends, and especially my wife for pushing me to finish—thank you, Dr. Robin Shaw. You're amazing! Lastly, my awesome children who believed in me to finish strong!

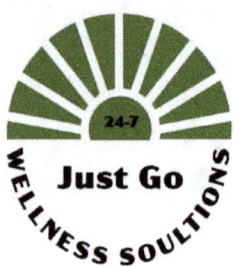

Wellness Resources

The Prostate Health Card is a resource for documenting prostate data, both the DRE and PSA. The card can be carried and easily accessed. Family, this makes knowing your prostate digits, doctor summary, and family medical history useful for early identification of trends. For Black people with high-risk, age thirty-five is the recommended age to get testing started. My family had four out of four get prostate cancer. Early detection saved three lives!

Use this book to pass along prostate awareness and family history to men in your life. Health is wealth, Family! Let's go!

Prostate Health Cards

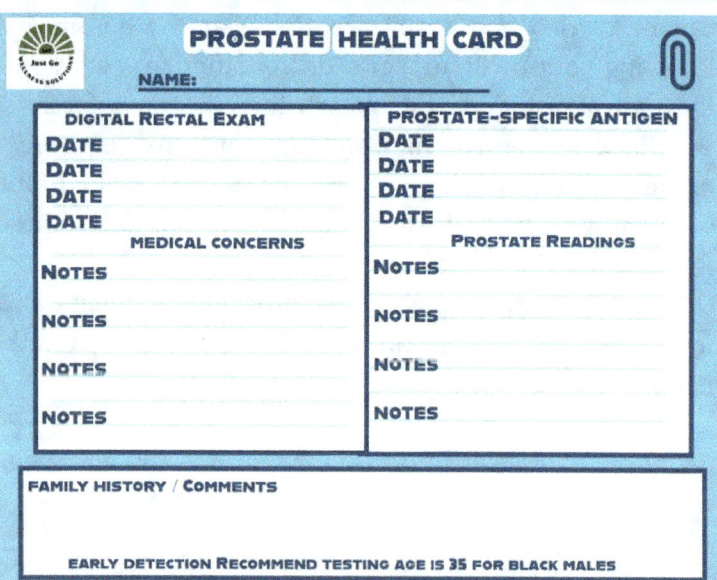

PROSTATE HEALTH CARD

NAME: _____

DIGITAL RECTAL EXAM	PROSTATE-SPECIFIC ANTIGEN
DATE _____	DATE _____
DATE _____	DATE _____
DATE _____	DATE _____
DATE _____	DATE _____
MEDICAL CONCERNS	PROSTATE READINGS
NOTES _____	NOTES _____
NOTES _____	NOTES _____
NOTES _____	NOTES _____
NOTES _____	NOTES _____

FAMILY HISTORY / COMMENTS

EARLY DETECTION RECOMMEND TESTING AGE IS 35 FOR BLACK MALES

PROSTATE HEALTH CARD

NAME: _____

DIGITAL RECTAL EXAM	PROSTATE-SPECIFIC ANTIGEN
DATE _____	DATE _____
DATE _____	DATE _____
DATE _____	DATE _____
DATE _____	DATE _____
MEDICAL CONCERNS	PROSTATE READINGS
NOTES _____	NOTES _____
NOTES _____	NOTES _____
NOTES _____	NOTES _____
NOTES _____	NOTES _____

FAMILY HISTORY / COMMENTS

EARLY DETECTION RECOMMEND TESTING AGE IS 35 FOR BLACK MALES

Wellness Resources

PROSTATE HEALTH CARD

NAME: _____

DIGITAL RECTAL EXAM	PROSTATE-SPECIFIC ANTIGEN
DATE	DATE
DATE	DATE
DATE	DATE
DATE	DATE
MEDICAL CONCERNS	**PROSTATE READINGS**
NOTES	NOTES
NOTES	NOTES
NOTES	NOTES
NOTES	NOTES

FAMILY HISTORY / COMMENTS

EARLY DETECTION RECOMMEND TESTING AGE IS 35 FOR BLACK MALES

PROSTATE HEALTH CARD

NAME: _____

DIGITAL RECTAL EXAM	PROSTATE-SPECIFIC ANTIGEN
DATE	DATE
DATE	DATE
DATE	DATE
DATE	DATE
MEDICAL CONCERNS	**PROSTATE READINGS**
NOTES	NOTES
NOTES	NOTES
NOTES	NOTES
NOTES	NOTES

FAMILY HISTORY / COMMENTS

EARLY DETECTION RECOMMEND TESTING AGE IS 35 FOR BLACK MALES

Peeling Back the Onion on Prostate Cancer 59

PROSTATE HEALTH CARD

NAME: _____

DIGITAL RECTAL EXAM
DATE _____
DATE _____
DATE _____
DATE _____

MEDICAL CONCERNS
NOTES _____
NOTES _____
NOTES _____
NOTES _____

PROSTATE-SPECIFIC ANTIGEN
DATE _____
DATE _____
DATE _____
DATE _____

PROSTATE READINGS
NOTES _____
NOTES _____
NOTES _____
NOTES _____

FAMILY HISTORY / COMMENTS

EARLY DETECTION RECOMMEND TESTING AGE IS 35 FOR BLACK MALES

PROSTATE HEALTH CARD

NAME: _____

DIGITAL RECTAL EXAM
DATE _____
DATE _____
DATE _____
DATE _____

MEDICAL CONCERNS
NOTES _____
NOTES _____
NOTES _____
NOTES _____

PROSTATE-SPECIFIC ANTIGEN
DATE _____
DATE _____
DATE _____
DATE _____

PROSTATE READINGS
NOTES _____
NOTES _____
NOTES _____
NOTES _____

FAMILY HISTORY / COMMENTS

EARLY DETECTION RECOMMEND TESTING AGE IS 35 FOR BLACK MALES

Wellness Resources

PROSTATE HEALTH CARD

NAME: _____

DIGITAL RECTAL EXAM
- DATE _____
- DATE _____
- DATE _____
- DATE _____

MEDICAL CONCERNS
- NOTES _____
- NOTES _____
- NOTES _____
- NOTES _____

PROSTATE-SPECIFIC ANTIGEN
- DATE _____
- DATE _____
- DATE _____
- DATE _____

PROSTATE READINGS
- NOTES _____
- NOTES _____
- NOTES _____
- NOTES _____

FAMILY HISTORY / COMMENTS

EARLY DETECTION RECOMMEND TESTING AGE IS 35 FOR BLACK MALES

PROSTATE HEALTH CARD

NAME: _____

DIGITAL RECTAL EXAM
- DATE _____
- DATE _____
- DATE _____
- DATE _____

MEDICAL CONCERNS
- NOTES _____
- NOTES _____
- NOTES _____
- NOTES _____

PROSTATE-SPECIFIC ANTIGEN
- DATE _____
- DATE _____
- DATE _____
- DATE _____

PROSTATE READINGS
- NOTES _____
- NOTES _____
- NOTES _____
- NOTES _____

FAMILY HISTORY / COMMENTS

EARLY DETECTION RECOMMEND TESTING AGE IS 35 FOR BLACK MALES

Prostate Health Recorder

Prostate Health Recorder

Family Medical History Recorder

Family Medical History Recorder

www.ingramcontent.com/pod-product-compliance
Lightning Source LLC
Chambersburg PA
CBHW050226100526
44585CB00017BA/2066